FIRST AID AND HEALTH CARE FOR CATS

Charles T.P. Bell
M.A. Vet. M.B., MRCVS

BERKLEY BOOKS, NEW YORK

This Berkley book contains the complete
text of the original edition.

FIRST AID AND HEALTH CARE FOR CATS

A Berkley Book / published by arrangement with
Pecos Press

PRINTING HISTORY
Pecos Press edition published 1990
Berkley edition / June 1991

ISBN: 0-425-13128-9

A BERKLEY BOOK ® TM 757,375
Berkley Books are published by The Berkley Publishing Group,
200 Madison Avenue, New York, New York 10016.
The name "BERKLEY" and the "B" logo
are trademarks belonging to Berkley Publishing Corporation.

PRINTED IN THE UNITED STATES OF AMERICA

10 9 8 7 6 5 4 3

Contents

Preface

It is my wish that no animal ever be confronted
with a "life or death" situation. However, accidents
do happen all too frequently. If your cat does suffer
an injury, you must make several decisions in a
very short period of time. Often, your choices will
affect your pet's overall well-being. *First Aid &
Health Care for Cats* was written to help you make
the right decisions.

No book can take the place of your veterinarian. In
the time of a crisis, the best chance for a favorable
outcome is to get your cat to your veterinarian as
quickly as possible. You should not waste time
trying to diagnose or to treat your pet's injury.
However, there are some basic steps that you can
take that might stabilize the animal, reducing the
chance of further damage and complications. These
are the procedures advocated in this book.

First Aid & Health Care for Cats works as a bridge
between your veterinarian and you. The two of you
are partners that share the same goal: maintaining
the good health of your cat. Reaching this goal is the
best way to ensure that your cat will enjoy a long,
happy life. The book can also help prepare you to
make the right choices for decisions that, hopefully,
you will never have to make.

The book is divided into three parts.

Part I–Health Care

Part I outlines the various components of a
general health care program. These
components are important to the main-
tenance of the overall good health of
your cat. A healthy cat is in the best
position to fight off diseases and the
effects of injuries. In addition, proper
health care for your pet will reduce the
chance of the animal transmitting a
parasite or disease to other members of
your family.

Part II–First Aid

This section gives the first aid procedures
that should be taken in many of the
most common emergency situations.
The steps described emphasize common sense, simplicity and your own
safety.

Each chapter begins with a short overview
that gives background information
about the emergency. Next are the
common signs that you are likely to see.
These are followed by the proper steps
to take. Just as important as telling you
what to do, the book indicates what you
should NOT do; it informs you of the
common mistakes that people often
make. Most chapters end by advising
you to take your injured pet to your

veterinarian; Chapter 21 details the correct manner to do this.

The layout of each chapter facilitates quick and easy use. In the time of a crisis, you will not have to waste time searching for the proper steps to take.

Part III–After the Emergency

Your veterinarian may ask you to take an active role on the recuperative process. This section instructs you how to administer medicine, check devices used for healing and deal with various issues associated with surgery.

Writing a book is a difficult task. Without the help and guidance of many individuals, this project would not have been completed. I would like to thank all of the reviewers (both the veterinarians and the non-veterinarians) for their comments. They forced me to factor out my own medical biases as well as to keep the material readily accessible to the intended audience. A special debt of gratitude goes to Alice Dworkin, whose advice pointed me in the right direction and comments kept me on course throughout the project.

I would also like to thank A. Christine MacMurray, Editor at the Animal Medical Center in New York City, for allowing me to access the the AMC's library while researching the material.

Lastly, Karen Fortgang of bookworks deserves credit for patiently guiding me through the various stages of production.

I would like to close with a word of warning. An injured animal can be a dangerous animal. A cat in pain may resist any handling and may lash out at you. You must be on guard and take precautions to protect yourself. If you are bitten or injured, you should seek medical attention.

About the Author

Charles T. P. Bell graduated from Cambridge University with a degree in Veterinary Medicine. Dr. Bell has practiced for several years in both the United Kingdom and the United States, specializing in small animals.

PART I

HEALTH
CARE

1 Preventive Medicine

Introduction

Preventive medicine is taking steps to prevent illness. By following a complete program, you help your cat maintain good health throughout its life. The most important aspects of a preventive medicine program are a well-balanced diet and regular veterinary examinations. Chapter 2 discusses nutrition (see page 15). Other components of preventive medicine are outlined below.

Going to Your Veterinarian

Regular trips to your veterinarian are crucial to the maintance of your cat's health. Your doctor can design a program geared specifically for your cat. Periodic examinations will allow the veterinarian to monitor your cat's progress and adjust the program as needed. In addition, your doctor will know of special issues that apply to your geographic location (such as the length of flea and tick season, the prevalence of certain diseases and the local ordinances that may pertain to pets).

You should visit your veterinarian for a number of reasons.

- It is easier to prevent a disease than to treat it. Your cat is better off if steps are taken to prevent an illness rather than if steps are needed to treat one. Some diseases cannot be treated (rabies being the most notorious).

- It is less expensive to prevent a disease than to treat it. Vaccinations may seem expensive, but they are much cheaper than a cure for an illness. The money spent on preventive medicine is like buying insurance against disease; it is the best insurance policy available for your pet.

- Your cat may not be the only one who gets sick. Some of the diseases that threaten your cat can be transmitted to humans and to other animals. Taking steps to keep your cat disease-free is important to the overall health of the entire family.

Your first trip to your veterinarian should be soon after obtaining your cat or kitten. This is the best time to begin a complete health program. After the first series of visits, your cat should be examined by your veterinarian at least once each year. In addition, you should have a test for worms performed every 6 months to 1 year, depending on your area.

When going to your veterinarian

- Take a recent fecal sample (also known as a stool sample). It should be less than 24 hours old; it will be used to check for worms and other intestinal parasites.

- Transport your cat in a catbox. There may be several animals at the clinic. You must be able to protect your cat as well as keep it under control.
- Try to remember any recent unusual behavior exhibited by your cat. Give the veterinarian as many details as you can.

Vaccinations

Vaccinations are powerful tools that stimulate the immune system, the natural line of defense against disease. Once a virus or bacteria has been introduced and fought off, the immune system remembers it and develops a mechanism to fight it in the future. A vaccine is made from the same agent that causes a disease, but the agent is altered so that it is harmless. The immune system, however, cannot tell the difference between the real agent and the vaccine. This allows the system to build up a defense to the disease without being subjected to it.

Most vaccinations are given when your cat is young. Kittens should receive 2 to 4 shots a few weeks apart. Staging the shots allows your kitten to gradually build up adequate immunity. Until it has received all of them, your kitten may not be fully protected. Annual booster vaccinations are needed to keep the immune system strong.

Diseases Prevented by Vaccinations

- Feline Leukemia—This is the most dangerous disease, accounting for the most disease-related deaths of cats. The virus is linked to many serious illnesses including leukemia, cancer and anemia. It can also lead to a suppressed immune system. By breaking down the natural defense, it may result in the development of such secondary problems as chronic gum infection, fever, miscarried pregnancies and kidney problems.

Feline leukemia can exhibit the "time bomb" effect. As such, a cat may be infected for many years before it will show any clinical signs of illness. Throughout this period, it may be able to transmit the virus to other cats. This disease can be prevented by an initial series of vaccinations followed by annual booster shots.

- Rabies—This is one of the most feared diseases; there is no cure. Rabies attacks the brain and the nervous system. The most common way that rabies is transmitted is through bites from infected wild animals. These often are raccoons, foxes, skunks, bats and stray dogs and cats.

Your kitten should have its first rabies vaccination at the age of 3 months.

After that, the vaccination can be given once a year or every 3 years. Your veterinarian will advise you on the best vaccine for your cat.

If your cat is bitten by an animal that you suspect may have rabies, go to your veterinarian immediately. Your cat may need an additional booster shot to strengthen its immune system and may need to be quarantined for observation.

People can also contract rabies. Anyone bitten by an animal should seek medical attention immediately.

• Feline Distemper—This attacks the intestinal tract and can cause severe diarrhea, vomiting and dehydration. Despite treatment, this disease frequently results in death.

A distemper vaccination usually includes vaccines for the feline calici virus and the feline herpes virus, which are the most common sources of respiratory disease in cats. Symptoms of respiratory disease include sneezing, conjunctivitis, debilitation and fever. They may permanently damage the respiratory system and can be life threatening.

Neutering

Neutering is the removal of the reproductive glands, preventing a cat from breeding. While this helps control the cat population, it has medical and behavioral benefits as well. Neutering does not alter the personality of your cat.

- Males—Neutering of males is known as altering or castration; it is the removal of the testicles. The most common time to have a male altered is around the age of 6 months.

Advantages of Altering

- Prevents unwanted pregnancies and kittens
- Often causes cat to be less aggressive (less likely to fight)
- Less likely to wander off (reducing its chance of being hit by car)
- Less likely to spray in the house. (Spraying is the type of urination used to mark territory.)
- Urine odor greatly reduced

Disadvantages of Altering

- Cannot breed
- Has to have an operation, requiring anesthesia

- May tend to gain weight (easily controlled by adjusting diet)

- Females—Neutering of females is known as spaying. This is the removal of the ovaries and uterus. The most common time to have a female spayed is around the age of 6 months.

Advantages of Spaying

- Prevents unwanted pregnancies and kittens
- Greatly reduces the risk of breast cancer, if performed early in life
- Eliminates the risk of pyometra, a very serious disease that involves the production of pus in the uterus
- Eliminates annoying behavior associated with going into "heat", such as repeated crying

Disadvantage of Spaying

- Cannot breed
- Has to have an operation, requiring anesthesia
- May tend to gain weight (easily controlled by adjusting diet)

Unless you plan to breed your cat, you should elect to have it neutered. The risk is very low (especially for a young cat) and outweighed by the medical benefits.

Parasites

There are a number of parasites that can affect your cat. These include worms, fleas, ticks, mites and mange. They are discussed in Chapter 3 (see page 25).

Environment

Cats are fastidious animals; they constantly clean themselves and prefer a clean environment. They also like privacy; the litter box should be placed in a secluded location that is separate from the feeding area. You should change the kitty litter and clean the bedding at least once a week. Stools in the litter box should be removed every day; it is advisable to wear gloves when doing so. These steps will decrease the chances that your cat or your family will contract parasites or diseases.

Skin Care

Good skin care helps prevent skin problems. These are usually difficult to treat and can lead to infection if a cat constantly bites or scratches itself. Once a cat has had a skin problem, it is often prone to contracting another.

All cats should be regularly brushed. Long-haired cats should be brushed every day. This removes mats and knots and reduces the chance of hairballs, clumps of ingested hair. In addition, regular brushing allows you to closely examine your cat, increasing the chance of early detection of problems. You should use a comb and brush designed specifically for cats.

Other steps may be required; your veterinarian can best advise you on how to care for your cat. Some suggestions are listed below.

- Diet supplements—There are several food supplements that can help your cat's skin. Any supplement should be designed for cats. Oversupplementation can be harmful; check with your doctor before beginning to use one.

- Fleas—Fleas should be treated quickly. They cause the cat to scratch and can lead to skin infection. Fleas are discussed in greater detail in Chapter 3 (see page 30).

Care of Teeth and Gums

The care of teeth and gums is becoming increasingly recognised as important for general good health. Cats with dental problems may develop bad breath and may go off their food. Poor dental care may lead to inflamed and infected gums, which in turn may result in loss of teeth. There is a chance that an infection will enter the bloodstream where it may affect internal organs such as the kidneys. Bad teeth and gums are especially debilitating for older animals. Consult with your veterinarian as to what steps you should take to foster good teeth and gums.

Example of Complete Health Program

The following is an example of a complete health program for your cat. Many variables need to be factored into this program. These include type of cat, type of vaccine, climate, local laws and other regional issues. These factors can change from time to time. As such, your veterinarian is in the best position to design a program that is suited to the specific needs of your cat. The two of you should work together to set it up.

Kitten

- Soon after acquisition
  - Complete physical by your veterinarian

- 8 to 10 weeks
  - Distemper vaccination
  - Fecal test
  - Feline leukemia test
  - Worming

- 10 to 12 weeks
  - Distemper vaccination
  - Feline leukemia vaccination
  - Worming

- 12 to 16 weeks
    - Rabies vaccination
    - Distemper vaccination
    - Feline leukemia vaccination

- 24 weeks
    - Feline leukemia vaccination

Adult

- Daily
    - Brush/comb out cat
    - Supplement food, if necessary (check with your veterinarian)

- Weekly
    - Weigh cat

- 6 Months
    - Fecal test
    - Worming

- Yearly
    - General exam by your veterinarian
    - Rabies vaccination
    - Distemper vaccination
    - Feline leukemia vaccination
    - Fecal test
    - Worming
    - Geriatric work-up (older cats only)

Summary

- Preventive medicine is a crucial concern for the health of not only your cat but also your entire family.
- You should visit your veterinarian soon after acquiring your kitten or cat.
- Your veterinarian should examine your cat at least once a year.
- Vaccinations help the immune system to fight off various diseases.
- Unless you plan to breed your cat, you should have it altered or spayed.
- Care of teeth and gums is an essential part of preventive medicine.

2   Nutrition

Introduction

Excellent health begins with good nutrition. The
keys to good nutrition are plenty of fresh water and
a well-balanced diet consisting of a high quality
food.

Fresh Water

It is crucial that your cat always has access to fresh,
clean water. Without sufficient water, it may dehydrate, leading to a wide variety of problems. It is a
good idea to make water available in several areas
in your home and to change the water daily. Adequate water is especially important for older cats.

What to Feed

A well-balanced diet begins with the correct food. It
is best to use a quality commercial diet which can be
bought at supermarkets, at pet stores and from
your veterinarian. Commercial food companies have
spent years and millions of dollars on the perfection
of their foods. The result is that these foods provide
the best mix of nutrients and flavor. A home-made
diet can be well-balanced, but it will probably be
more expensive than a good commercial brand and
it may leave out important nutrients.

The food that you select should be designed specifically for cats. Even though it is generally less

expensive than cat food, dog food should not be given to cats. Cats have a significantly different set of nutritional requirements; they need a higher level of protein. Dog food is not well-balanced for cats.

Once you have decided on a type of food, do not change often. A cat's digestive system does not adapt well to sudden change. This often causes diarrhea. However, your cat would probably enjoy a wide variety of tastes. Many types of cat food come in different flavors.

Milk is not necessary for a cat's health. Some do not tolerate it and it is a common cause of diarrhea. But if your cat enjoys the taste and does not suffer any ill effects, milk can be given.

It is important to clean the water and feed bowls on a regular basis. Also food must be stored properly after it has been opened; instructions for this are usually written on the package. Any food that appears moldy or has a rancid odor should be discarded.

Types of Food Available

There are three main types of cat food available today.

- Dry
    - Low moisture (stays fresh in feed bowl)
    - Inexpensive

- Convenient

- Semi-Moist
    - Stays fresh in bowl for several hours
    - Often not good as a total diet; best as a supplement

- Canned Meat
    - Very palatable and nutritious
    - Usually the most expensive
    - Will not stay fresh very long in bowl

Several factors should be considered when selecting the best food for your cat. A few are listed below.

- Age of cat (Kitten, adult or older cat)
- Cat's quirks (will eat anything or very finicky)
- Cost of food

Special Diets

There are special diets available to assist in the treatment or management of important medical conditions, such as kidney disease, heart disease, FUS & other urinary problems, obesity and several others. Your veterinarian can determine if your cat has a condition that may respond to dietary modification and recommend the best product. While many "lite" foods are available to help promote weight loss, you should not make a change in diet without first consulting your veterinarian.

How Much to Feed

Most cat foods have a feeding chart on the package. However, this chart should be used only as a rough guideline. Each cat is different; some need more food than others. By experimenting with various portions of food, you will eventually determine the best amount for your cat. Your veterinarian should be consulted on this matter, as well.

How Often to Feed

A guideline for how often to feed is below. Again, not all cats are the same. Your veterinarian can help you determine the proper feeding schedule.

- Up to 4 months—4 times a day
- 4 to 6 months—3 times a day
- 6 months and beyond—2 times a day

Most adult cats do better on 2 feedings a day rather than only one. Some will eat their food so fast that they make themselves sick. For a cat such as this, you might feed it the same amount of food but split the portions up into smaller quantities and feed more often. In addition, you may want to leave out a dry snack food throughout the day. These snack foods, however, are not designed to be the sole source of nutrients; they are not well-balanced. If your cat snacks to the point that it loses interest in its main diet, you should limit the amount of food between meals.

Controlling Weight

Ideal weight varies with each individual cat. Your veterinarian and you can determine the best weight for your cat. Once this has been established, you can help your cat maintain that weight through periodic evaluations. Two methods are outlined below.

Measuring by touch

- Stand the cat up.
- Place hands on opposite sides of the rib cage. Cat is overweight if you cannot feel the ribs at all.

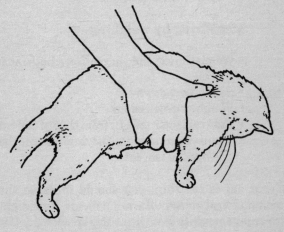

- Feel for the neural spines of the vertebrae in the lower back. Cat is underweight if these are readily detectable.

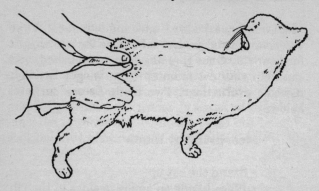

- Cat is ideal if you can just feel each rib and there is good muscle depth on either side of the back bone.

Measuring by weighing

- Weigh the cat and yourself on a bathroom scale.
- Set the cat down.
- Weigh yourself alone.
- Subtract your weight from that of the cat and you combined. The difference is the weight of the cat.

If your cat is too thin, you should increase the amount of food given at the main meals. You might also supplement its diet with a dry snack food. If it still does not gain weight, your cat should be examined by your veterinarian. An older cat that is losing weight should be taken to your doctor. If your cat is overweight, take steps to help it lose weight.

Losing Weight

Excess weight is the most common nutritional problem of cats. Almost a third of the cats in the United States suffer from obesity. An overweight cat is a walking time bomb. Obesity contributes to such long-term illnesses as heart disease, diabetes and certain forms of cancer. In addition, lugging around the extra weight is uncomfortable (especially in hot weather). You can help your cat lose weight.

Steps for weight loss

- Reduce amount of food given per day by a third.
- Change regular food to a special diet food.
- Eliminate all snacks.

Dieting for cats can be dangerous, just as it can be for people. You should consult your veterinarian before taking any step that may cause your cat to lose weight.

Food Supplements

There are several types of supplements that are helpful to your cat's health. However, not all are beneficial. It is important to stick to the recommended dosage. Oversupplementing can be harmful.

- Vitamins—Kittens and older cats often need more nutrients than an adult. Vitamins designed specifically for cats can meet this need. However, consult your doctor before using them.

• Snack foods—Discussed in "How Often to Feed" section. These can be good as long as your cat does not lose interest in the main meals.

• Bones—These are not good for cats. A swallowed bone is not easily digestible and can lead to stomach and intestinal problems. It might have to be taken out by surgery.

• Oils—Certain oils can be added to the regular food. Oils help make the coat healthy and shiny. They can also make the food taste better. There are several products available through veterinarians and pet stores that make good oil supplements. Small amounts of corn oil and olive oil (1/4 to 1/2 teaspoon a day) also are good. If your cat starts producing soft stools, reduce the amount of oil given.

Tablescraps

Tablescraps are not good for a cat. They often upset the stomach, causing vomiting and diarrhea. In addition, they are the leading cause of obesity and foster annoying behavior, such as begging.

Summary

- Always have clean, fresh water available.
- Choose a commercial cat food that provides a complete, balanced diet.
- Do not change type of food often.
- Adjust the amount of food given to suit your cat's needs.
- Adjust the number of times of feeding a day to suit your cat's needs.
- Regularily check your cat's weight.
- Supplements can be good for your cat.
- Do not feed your cat tablescraps.

3   Parasites

Introduction

A parasite is an organism that lives off of another organism to the detriment of the host. A number of parasites affect cats. Besides being debilitating to animals, some can affect people. As soon as a cat is detected to have parasites, it should be treated promptly and thoroughly.

Worms

There are many types of worms. Some of the more common are discussed below.

- Roundworm—Looks like small spaghetti. Can cause vomiting, diarrhea, weight loss and lack of growth (in kittens).

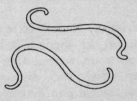

  If cat is heavily infected, worms may be seen in vomit or stools. Transmitted through ingestion of soiled material, feces or milk (from the mother when kittens are suckling). Can be transmitted to humans through ingestion of soiled material and feces.

- Tapeworm—Looks like rice grains attached to the anus. Can be fairly mobile and may move around like a slow motion slinky.

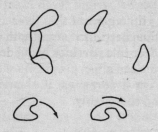

Usually does not show any clinical signs, but can cause diarrhea and weight loss in some cases. Transmitted by ingestion of an infected flea or eating wild animals such as mice and rats. Can infect humans if an infected flea is swallowed (cannot be transmitted directly from the cat).

- Hookworm—Usually 1/2 to 1 inch in length and in the shape of a hook. Smaller than roundworms. Can cause vomiting, weight loss, emaciation, anemia, pneumonia and diarrhea. Sometimes causes the production of dark, tarry feces. Transmitted by penetration through the skin or ingestion. Can also affect humans.

There are several signs to look for if you think that your cat might have worms.

Signs of Worms

- Vomiting and/or diarrhea
- Pot belly abdomen (mainly in kittens)
- Loss of weight (even if eating more food than normal)
- Spaghetti-like particles in vomit or feces
- Rice-like particles around the anus

What to Do

- Collect a fecal sample (also known as a stool sample).
- Take the sample and your cat to your veterinarian for an examination.

Your doctor will test the stool sample. If the tests are positive, your cat will be treated with an injection and/or oral medicine. Most successful treatment requires two stages. The first stage will kill the existing worms but not their eggs. The second kills the recently hatched worms before they can breed. The timing between the two is crucial; follow your veterinarian's instructions diligently.

You can minimize the chance of contracting worms.

Steps of Prevention

- Clean the litter box often. Wear gloves when doing so.
- Do not let your cat eat mice or rats.
- Have a stool sample tested every 6 months.
- Treat for fleas as needed.

Other Intestinal Parasites

Besides worms, other parasites afflict the intestinal tract. Signs, treatment and prevention of these are similar to that of worms.

- Coccidia—Tiny parasite that lives in the intestinal tract; seen only through a microscope. Can cause diarrhea (occasionally with blood), weight loss and dehydration. Transmitted by ingestion of fecal-contaminated material.

- Giardia—Also a microscopic parasite living in the intestines. Similar symptoms and characteristics to those of coccidia. Can be transmitted to people.

- Toxoplasma—Microscopic parasite that migrates through body tissue. It can produce a wide variety of symptoms and can affect virtually any organ. But it is often carried without showing any clinical signs.

  Toxoplasma can infect people. Those most at risk are people who have impaired immune systems, such as those undergoing chemotherapy or those with AIDS. In addition, it has been known to migrate through the placenta of pregnant women and cause birth defects or miscarriages.

While the parasite is usually transmitted by eating undercooked meat, it can also be transmitted through the ingestions of cat feces or fecal contaminated food. Infected cats excrete the parasite in the form of cysts in their feces. In order to become infective to people, the cysts must mature. This process can take from 12 hours to 5 days after excretion of feces.

There are steps to prevent toxoplasmosis.

- The cat should have a blood test to check for antibodies against the parasite.
- The cat should have frequent fecal tests; your veterinarian can help you set up a schedule.
- Clean the litter box twice a day.
- Wear rubber gloves.
  - Pregnant woman and immuno-suppressed people should not clean the litter box.
- People who think that they may be at risk should check with their physician.

Ringworm

Contrary to its name, ringworm is not a worm; it is

a fungus that causes skin disease. It is transmitted by contact with an infected cat or its environment. Common sites of ringworm are animal shelters and other locations where large groups of animals are kept. Kittens are most commonly affected; ringworm can infect people as well, particularly small children.

Signs of Ringworm

- Hair loss in patches
- Lesions around eyes, ears, head and feet
- Scaling and crusting of skin
- Excessive scratching

What to Do

- Transport to your veterinarian (see page 123).

Fleas

The most likely reason that a cat scratches itself is that it has fleas. Fleas are insects often seen running or jumping around an infected animal. They feed by biting the animal and sucking its blood.

Fleas are harmful in two ways. First, they often cause skin infections. Flea bites itch; heavy scratching irritates the skin and makes the cat prone to infections. Some cats are allergic to flea bites. Thus, one bite alone can lead to a serious skin problem. Second, they feed on blood. When biting through the skin, they can transmit diseases into the bloodstream. Both of these problems can affect people, too. A heavy flea infestation can cause anemia, which can be fatal (especially for kittens).

Fleas thrive in warm weather. As such, they are a year-round problem in warm climates. While prevalent mainly during the summer months in cold climates, fleas can continue to live indoors if the temperature inside is constantly warm. They can infest even the cleanest home.

In order to control fleas, you must treat both the cat and the cat's environment. Fleas can move quickly and easily. If you treat the cat but not the home and yard, the problem will persist. Also, if you have more than one animal, you should treat them all at the same time.

There are a number of good products available for controlling fleas. Your veterinarian can tell you which products work best in your area.

Steps to Take to Control Fleas

- Use a flea and tick powder or spray designed for cats once a week. It is important to read the product label and to follow the instructions carefully; incorrect use can lead to poisoning. Small

kittens may need special treatment; check with your veterinarian.
- Use flea and tick collar. This will limit the number of fleas but may not totally control them. Check the neck once a week for any signs of skin reaction.
- Treat your home and yard with a top-quality flea control product.
- Clean the cat's bedding once a week.

Ticks

Ticks are large parasites that feed by sucking blood. They bury their heads in the skin (usually around the head, neck and ear areas) and are difficult to remove. Since they penetrate the skin, they can transmit diseases such as Lymes Disease. Lymes is a bacterial disease that can cause fever, lethargy, heart problems, kidney failure, meningitis and sore joints. It can affect people as well, but it is usually transmitted directly from the Deer Tick.

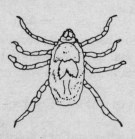

Tick season occurs in warm weather. During this time, you should examine your cat everytime it comes in from outside. If you see a tick, remove it at once.

Steps to Control Ticks

• Use a flea and tick collar.
• Use a flea and tick powder once a week.
• Examine the cat when it comes in from outside.

What to Do—Removing a Tick

• Spray a heavy dose of tick spray directly on the tick or cover it with strong alcohol. Be careful not to get any spray or alcohol into your cat's mouth, nose, eyes or ear canal.
• Wait 5 minutes.
• Pull tick off using a pair of tweezers. (Do not use your fingers; direct contact with a tick may increase the chance of you contracting a disease from it.)
   • Grasp tick as close to the skin as possible.

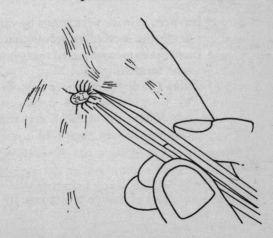

> - Pull using a steady, even pressure. Do not use a sudden jerk or twist.
> - Contact your veterinarian if you have any problems. The most common problem is leaving the head of the tick in the skin; this often leads to infection.

Ear Mites

Ear mites are tiny parasites that affect cats in two ways. First, they cause itching which, when alleviated by heavy scratching, can lead to ruptured blood vessels. Second, the mites cause the ear to secrete a thick waxy discharge that often clogs the ear canal. Both can lead to ear infection. Mites are transmitted by direct contact with infected animals; this often happens to kittens still in the litter and to outdoor cats.

Steps To Control Ear Mites

- Have cat or kitten examined by your veterinarian soon after acquisition.
- Have the ears examined if there is persistent scratching.
- Follow the directions for treatment given by your doctor. The proper way to administer ear medication is shown in Chapter 22 (see page 138).

Mange

The many varieties of mange are caused by mites

that burrow into the skin or that live in the hair or on the scalp. They are most often found around the head, neck, eyes or ears. They can cause a tremendous amount of scratching, making the cat susceptible to infection. Some forms of mange can be transmitted to people.

Signs of Mange

- Heavy scratching
- Loss of hair
- Dry, scaly skin over parts of the body
- Sores covering parts of the body.

What to Do

- Transport to your veterinarian (see page 123).

Summary

- It is not uncommon for a cat to have parasites.
- Parasites can be a health hazard to people.
- All parasites should be eradicated as soon as detected.
- Your cat should be checked for worms regularly.
- When controlling fleas, you must treat both the cat and the cat's environment.
- Successful flea treatment must be consistent and thorough.
- When removing a tick, contact your veterinarian if you leave the head of the

tick in your cat.
- Have your cat examined if there is persistent scratching.

4   The Older Cat

Introduction

As a cat ages, its body begins to lose its ability to fight off disease and to repair itself. An older cat can have an enjoyable and rewarding life, but this stage of life requires some adjustments. While this chapter gives you some ideas, your veterinarian is the best source of information and advice.

Aging

Every cat ages at a different rate. Some cats will show signs of aging at about 8 years, others may not until they are 14 or 15 years old.

Signs of an Older Cat

- Less active than usual
- Changes in normal habits, such as sleeping more
- Changes in personality
- More sensitive to extreme heat and cold

These are normal signs of aging and should not alarm you (unless there is a sudden change). But you should discuss them with your veterinarian on your next visit.

The immune system of an older cat is less effective, making it more susceptible to disease and illness. In addition, the body organs do not function as well in an older cat as they do in a younger one. Some cats begin to have problems with their kidneys, heart, liver or thyroid glands. If any of the signs listed below appear, your cat should be examined by your veterinarian.

Signs of Problems in an Older Cat

- Loss of weight
- Vomiting and diarrhea
- Loss of appetite
- Increased drinking and urinating
- Pain
- Difficulty standing
- Difficulty breathing
- Bumping into objects
- Blood in urine
- Coughing
- Drooling
- Reduced sense of hearing

Loss of weight is a common sign in a cat slowly developing a disease. It is a good idea to weigh your cat once a week as it gets older. This will allow you to monitor any gradual changes.

Nutrition

The nutritional needs of an older cat are different from those of one in the prime of life. As a cat loses some of its energy, its need for food reduces and its ability to digest food may be impaired. Without a change in its diet, your cat may become overweight. Obesity compounds problems related to aging.

Changing the type of food may be a good idea. Several foods geared for the needs of an older cat are available. In addition, there are foods designed for cats with specific problems, like heart disease, kidney disease and bladder stones. Adding a vitamin supplement designed for cats may also be beneficial.

Above all, you should provide enough clean, fresh water in several locations. Many older cats suffer from kidney problems or failure. The result is that more water than normal is released into the urine. Additional water is needed to replace the large amount voided by urinating. Low levels of water may lead to dehydration. This can damage many internal organs, cause the build up of toxic by-products and potentially develop into a life-threatening condition.

Check with your veterinarian before making any changes to your cat's diet or adding a supplement. Your doctor has your cat's medical background and can help you make the best decisions.

The Geriatric Work-Up

In older cats, many major problems and diseases develop slowly. Early diagnosis greatly increases the chance of successful treatment and management of problems. To help catch them early, many veterinarians are now offering a geriatric work-up.

The geriatric work-up is a series of tests and exams that may show that a problem is developing. With the results, your veterinarian can advise you on steps to take that will maximize your cat's good health and life expectancy. The work-up can become a regular component of your annual visit.

The following is an example of a very thorough work-up illustrating the possibilities of modern veterinary medicine. The actual work-up chosen for your cat can vary tremendously depending on the result of the physical examination and your cat's medical history.

An Example of a Geriatric Work-Up

- Complete physical examination
- X-ray of chest
- X-ray of the abdomen
- Complete blood test
- Thyroid test
- Urine test
- Electrocardiogram

Summary

- Older cats can enjoy life and be happy.
- Signs of aging are not serious unless there are other signs of problems.
- Loss of weight is a good clue to something being wrong.
- Changing your cat's diet might be a good idea.
- Access to clean, fresh water in several locations is imperative for older cats.
- Do not switch to a special food or a supple-

ment for an older cat before checking with your veterinarian.

- A geriatric work-up once a year may help head off problems.

PART II

FIRST AID

5   Essential Procedures

Overview

There are several basic procedures that you should know. These will allow you to monitor your cat's health between visits to the veterinarian.

Weighing Your Cat

Obesity is a common problem among cats. Regular weighing will help you control your cat's weight.

What to Do

- Weigh the cat and yourself on a bathroom scale.
- Set the cat down.
- Weigh yourself alone.
- Subtract your weight from that of the cat and you combined. The difference is the weight of your cat.

Taking a Temperature

Normal temperature is 101 to 102.5 degrees Fahrenheit. Use a rectal thermometer.

What to Do

- Shake the thermometer down to about 95 or 96 degrees.
- Lubricate the thermometer with petro-

leum jelly.
- Have somebody hold the cat.
- Raise and hold the tail.
- Insert into the anus. Use a gentle twisting motion. Insert about half of the thermometer.

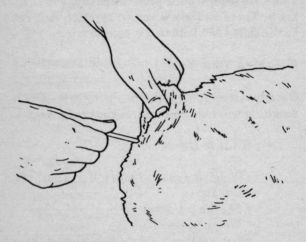

- Keep hold of both the thermometer and the tail.
- Leave in for 30 seconds to 1 minute.
- Pull out, wipe clean and read.

What NOT to Do

- Do NOT let go of the thermometer while inserted in your cat.
- Do NOT attempt to take a temperature if your cat struggles.
- Do NOT take temperature orally.

Taking a Pulse

The normal pulse rate is 150-240 beats per minute. There are two easy ways to take a pulse.

What to Do

Hand On Chest

- Grasp the chest just behind the elbows with one hand while supporting the cat with the other.

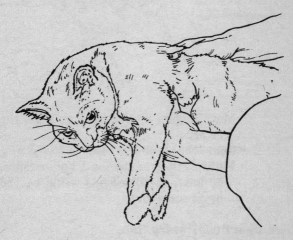

- Move the hand until you feel the heart beat.
- Count the number of beats in 20 seconds.
- Multiply that number by 3. For instance, 50 beats in 20 seconds would be 150 beats per minute.

Hand on the Femoral Artery

- Place fingers on inside of back leg where it joins the body.

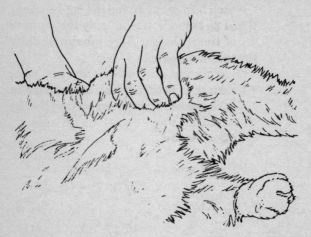

- Move fingers around until you feel the artery.
- Count the number of beats in 20 seconds.
- Multiply that number by 3. For instance, 60 beats in 20 seconds would be 180 beats per minute.

Taking a Respiratory Rate

The normal respiratory rate is between 10 and 30 breaths per minute. This rate can be much higher during and after playing. The number of breaths per minute can be measured by watching the chest or by placing a tissue in front of the nose.

What to Do

Watch the Chest

- Watch how many times the cat breathes
  in 20 seconds. (Count only the number
  of times the cat fully inhales or fully
  exhales, not both.)
- Multiply that number by 3. For instance,
  8 breaths in 20 seconds is a rate of 24
  per minute.

Using a Tissue

- Hold a tissue in front of the nose.

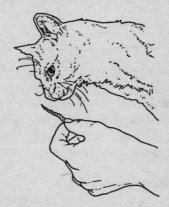

- Count how many times it moves in 20
  seconds.
- Multiply that number by 3. For instance,
  if the tissue moves 6 times in 20 seconds, the rate is 18 per minute.

6   CPR: Life Saving Procedures

Overview

CPR (cardiopulmonary resuscitation) consists of two procedures that may save the life of your cat: mouth-to-nose respiration and heart massage. While they may be life-saving, they can also be detrimental; you may aggravate your cat's condition if you do not properly administer these procedures.

You should not attempt either of these unless you encounter two conditions. First, do not attempt CPR unless proper veterinary care is unavailable. If you can get to a veterinarian quickly, your cat will have a better chance of survival than if you try CPR yourself. Second, do not attempt either procedure unless it is obvious that your cat will die if you do nothing. In a horrible situation such as that, doing something is better than nothing at all.

If you attempt CPR and do not successfully revive your cat, do not think that you have failed. Trained professionals, using state-of-the-art techniques and drugs, often cannot save a cat. You can only do your best.

Mouth-To-Nose Respiration

After a serious accident, your cat may stop breathing. If you cannot detect any respiratory signs and proper veterinary care is too far away, you should try to get the lungs started again by giving mouth-to-nose respiration.

What to Do

- Clear the airway.
    - Pull the tongue forward.

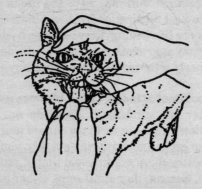

                    - Remove any material that may be blocking the throat.
- Close mouth firmly.

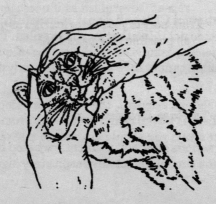

- Place your mouth over the nose of the cat.

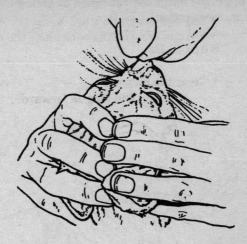

- Blow into nose until the chest expands
  fully (usually 1/2 to 1 second).
- Take mouth from nose, allowing the cat
  to exhale.
- Repeat the procedure for 10 seconds.
- Check cat for breathing on its own. If not,
  repeat (several times if necessary).
- Transport to your veterinarian as quickly
  as possible (see page 123).

Heart Massage

After a serious accident, the heart may stop beating. If there is no pulse and proper veterinary care is too far away, you should attempt to massage the heart.

What to Do

- Lay the cat on its side.
- Put one hand on the back along the spine.

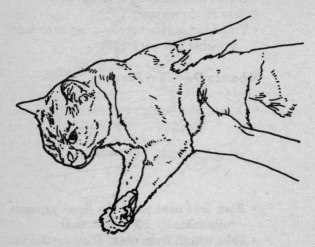

- Grasp the chest with the other hand.
- Push in firmly but gently. (Too much force may break the ribs.)
- Repeat rapidly for 15 seconds.
- Check for pulse.
- Repeat, if necessary.
- Transport to your veterinarian as quickly as possible (see page 123).

CPR (Cardiopulmonary Resuscitation)

CPR is the combination of giving mouth-to-nose respiration and massaging the heart.

What to Do—One Person

- Do mouth-to-nose for 10 seconds.
- Massage heart for 15 seconds.
- Check for breathing and a pulse rate.
- Repeat, if necessary.
- Transport to your veterinarian as soon as possible (see page 123).

What to Do—Two Persons

- One person gives mouth-to-nose.

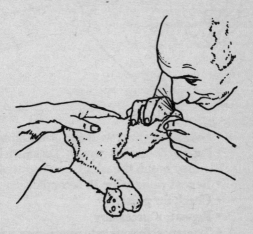

- The other massages the heart.
- Continue for 10-15 seconds.
- Check for breathing and a pulse rate.
- Repeat, if necessary.
- Transport to your veterinarian as soon as possible (see page 123).

Crucial Point to Remember

Do NOT attempt mouth-to-nose, heart massage or
CPR unless....

- Proper veterinary care is not available.
- It is obvious that your cat will not survive
  if you do nothing.

7 Unidentified Emergency

Overview

It is possible that you might encounter an emergency situation in which you have no idea as to what might be wrong or what caused the problem. In an instance such as this, you should transport your cat to your veterinarian as quickly as possible. Your doctor will probably ask you numerous questions while examining your pet. You should try to provide as much information as possible.

Signs of Unidentified Emergency

- Cat collapsed or prostrate
- Unattributed unusual behavior

What to Do

- Transport to your veterinarian (see page 123). While en route to the clinic, think back over the recent past. By reviewing your cat system by system, you might pick up some clues.

    #### General
    - Less alert than normal?
    - Less active than normal?
    - Change in appetite or drinking pattern?
    - Outside for unusual period of time?

- Access to any substances that may be poisonous, such as insecticides, antifreeze, medicines or mouse/rat poison?
- How long has there been a problem?

Respiratory
- Difficulty breathing?
- Coughing or wheezing?
- Discharge from nose?
- Rapid respiratory rate?

Gastrointestinal
- Vomiting or diarrhea?
- Change in diet?
- Eating things that it should not?
- Bleeding from mouth or gums?
- Broken teeth?

Cardiovascular
- Reduced tolerance to exercise?
- Change in color of gums?

Urogenital
- Straining to urinate?
- Urinating more frequently?
- Discharge from vulva or penis?

Neurological
- Change in behavior?
- Bumping into objects?
- Staring into space?
- Unstable posture or falling over?

Musculoskeletal
- Limping or lameness?
- Pain if touched in certain areas?
- Difficulty in climbing stairs?
- Difficulty in standing up after lying for a period of time?

Integument
- Cuts or bruises?
- Bleeding?
- Hair loss?
- Excessive scratching?
- Biting at certain areas?
- Dull coat?
- Dirt or unusual substance on coat?
- Split or broken toenails?

Ocular
- Sensitivity to light?
- Discharge from eyes?
- Third eyelid across?

What NOT to Do

- Do NOT waste time in attempting to diagnose your cat's condition. An unidentified emergency is often very serious. The key to survival may be reaching proper medical evaluation and treatment as fast as possible.

8   Hit by Car, Falls & Trauma

Overview

The two most common causes of trauma for a cat are being hit by a car and falling out of a window (the high rise syndrome). This often results in very serious injuries such as a crushed chest, broken bones, brain concussions, open and closed wounds, internal bleeding and internal organ damage. In addition, the cat usually goes into shock, in which case blood flow to the skin and many organs is shut down.

Use care when handling an injured animal. A cat in pain may resist any manipulation and can inflict considerable damage. Should you be scratched or bitten by a cat, seek medical attention immediately.

You may not see your cat get hit by a car or fall from a great height. But you may suspect it if you notice several signs.

Signs of Hit by Car, Falls and Trauma

- Difficulty breathing
- Scrapes and cuts
- Pain
- Limping or dragging a leg
- Cannot stand up properly

- Bleeding from nose
- Broken teeth or jaw
- Bruises
- Split toenails

What to Do—ABCs

A good sequence of steps for first aid is known as the ABCs.

A—Airway
B—Breathing
C—Circulation

If your cat shows no signs of life, transport to your veterinarian immediately (see page 123). If proper medical care is unavailable, attempt CPR (see page 51).

Airway

Airway first aid is clearing the airway tract so that the cat can breathe.

What To Do

- Pull the tongue out.

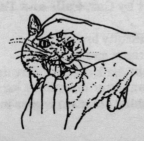

- Remove any blood or damaged tissue from the back of the mouth.

Breathing

Breathing first aid is ensuring that the cat is breathing properly.

> **If breathing OK, go to steps for Circulation (see page 66).**

> **If there is a wound penetrating the chest cavity, air can enter the chest around the lungs. This makes normal breathing difficult or impossible. You should try to make an airtight seal over the wound.**

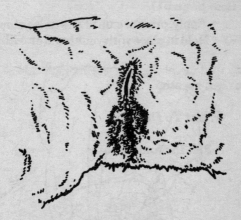

Sign of Air Entering through a Wound

• Sucking noise as air goes in and out

What to Do

• **Place cloth or plastic over the wound.**

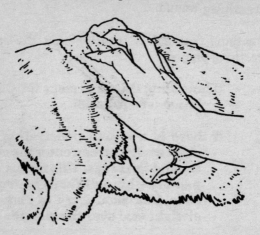

• **Apply pressure until the noise stops.**
• **Hold in place with your hand or with tape.**

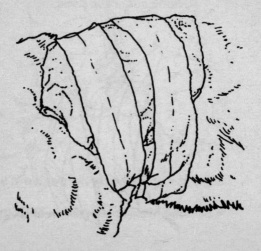

- **Do NOT hold or tape too tightly. This makes breathing too difficult.**
- **Do NOT pull out objects from a chest wound.**

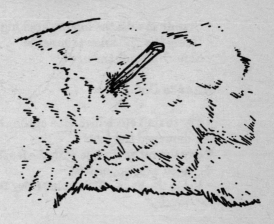

This may cause more damage. Place a bandage or plastic around any object sticking out of the chest.

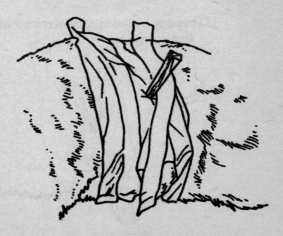

If the chest has been crushed, the cat will have difficulty breathing.

Signs of Crushed Chest

- Standing with the elbows sticking out
- Using the abdomen to breathe
- Stretching out the neck

What to Do

- Try to find out which side of the chest is damaged the least.
- Lay the cat on its side with the least damaged side uppermost.
- Raise the head. (This helps clear the airway.)

Circulation

Circulation first aid is controlling any bleeding.

If there is bleeding, control by applying pressure.

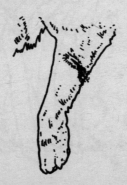

What to Do

- Wad up some cloth or gauze.
- Place it directly on the wound.

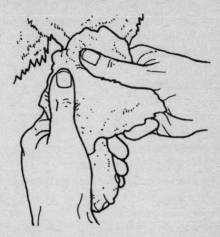

- Hold firmly but gently.

After ABCs

What to Do

- Transport to your veterinarian (see page 123).

What NOT to Do

- Do NOT assume that your cat is out of danger if it appears to be in good shape. It may have suffered internal damage. The full extent of the injury may not be apparent for several hours or even days. By then, your cat may be in critical condition.

9   Broken Legs, Sprains, Strains & Dislocations

Overview

Most broken bones (fractures) are caused by being hit by a car or falling from heights. Fractures can be divided into two main groups: open and closed. An open fracture is when a bone breaks and cuts through the skin; it can easily be infected. If the skin is not pierced, it is a closed fracture. A major goal of closed fracture first aid is to keep it from becoming an open fracture.

A sprain is a condition in which muscles or ligaments twist beyond normal limits. A strain is the excessive stretching of muscles and tendons. A bone popping out of a joint or socket is a dislocation. It is difficult to tell the difference between a closed fracture and a sprain, strain or dislocation. Thus, they should be handled in a similar manner until veterinary care is reached.

Use care when handling an injured animal. A cat in pain may resist any manipulation and can inflict considerable damage. If you are scratched or bitten by a cat, seek medical attention.

Signs of Breaks, Sprains, Strains & Dislocations

• Cracking or breaking sound at moment of

impact
- Change in size, shape or length of leg; may rest at a strange angle
- Standing on only three legs, the injured leg hanging limp
- Swelling around the injured area
- Pain
- Broken bone may be visible

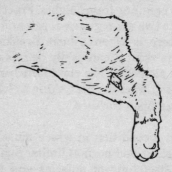

What to Do

- Move the injured leg as little as possible.
- If the bone is exposed, cover it with a light gauze or bandage.

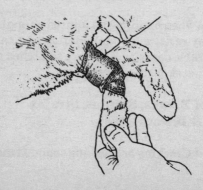

- Keep the cat as warm as possible; cover it
  with a blanket. (This will reduce the
  effects of shock.)
- Place a folded towel under the leg for support.

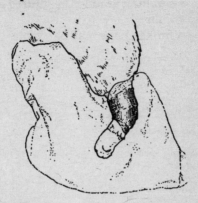

- Transport to your veterinarian (see page
  123).

What NOT to Do

- Do NOT attempt to splint the leg. The
  swelling makes it difficult to determine
  the exact location of the injury. A cat in
  pain will probably resist manipulation
  of the injured limb. Forced treatment is
  painful and may cause more damage.
  Use a folded towel to support the leg.

10   Wounds

Overview

A wound is a break in the continuity of tissue in any part of the body. Frequently, it is painful. You must exercise caution when handling a wounded animal. A cat in pain may bite or lash out. If you are bitten or scratched, seek medical attention.

There are two basic types of wounds: closed and open. With most wounds, there is a danger of infection. In addition, special steps should be taken if the wound is the result of a snake bite or insect sting.

Closed Wounds

A closed wound can be an abrasion or contusion (also known as a bruise); it is a wound where the skin remains unbroken. However, there may be significant internal damage that goes undetected. The injured skin may die and fall off a few days after the injury occurred; it may also become infected. The area affected is not always obvious and the extent of the damage may not be apparent for several days. A common cause of a closed wound is heavy friction on the skin or a blow from a blunt object.

Signs of a Closed Wound

- Pain

- Heat in a small area
- Skin scratched up
- Swelling

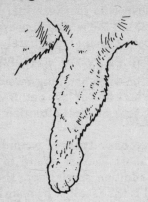

What to Do

- Bathe the area in cold water.
- Apply an ice pack. Use an icebag or place ice in a towel.

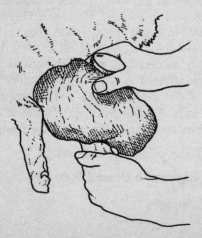

- If skin is scratched up, clean with 3% hydrogen peroxide or salt water (1 teaspoon salt to 1 pint warm water).
- Transport to your veterinarian (see page 123). If the wound appears serious, go to your doctor immediately. If not, go as soon as possible. All minor wounds should be checked by a veterinarian within 24 hours.

What NOT to Do

- Do NOT underestimate a closed wound. While it may look harmless, it can hide major internal damage. The full extent of the damage may not be apparent for several days. By then, your cat's condition may be very serious.

Open Wounds

An open wound is where the skin is broken, usually accompanied by significant bleeding. The loss of large amounts of blood can be life threatening. In addition, muscles, tendons, blood vessels and nerves may be severed and internal organs may be damaged. Since the outer layer of the body is open, dirt and bacteria can enter, leading to possible infection.

Signs of an Open Wound

- Pain
- Limping

- Excessive licking of certain areas
- Bleeding

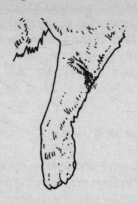

What to Do

- Use pressure to control the bleeding.
  - Wad up some clean cloth or gauze.
  - Place directly on the wound.
  - Hold firmly but gently.

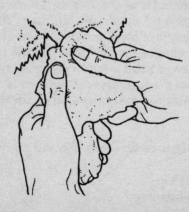

- **If the wound is minor, clean the wound.**
  - **Flush the wound with 3% hydrogen peroxide or salt water (1 teaspoon salt to 1 pint warm water).**

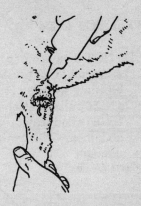

- **Dab clean with gauze or cloth. Do NOT rub. This hurts and may cause more damage.**

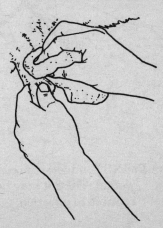

- Transport to your veterinarian (see page 123). A cat with a major wound should go to the doctor immediately. A minor wound should be checked within 24 hours.

What NOT to Do

- Do NOT delay transporting to your veterinarian. Use pressure to control the bleeding while en route.
- Do NOT pull out an object that has penetrated a body cavity such as the chest or abdomen. This might cause more damage.

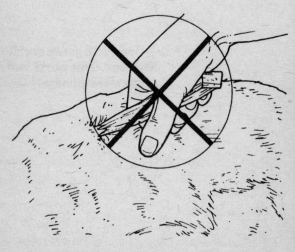

- Do NOT underestimate a small open wound. The cut may be deep and susceptible to infection.

Infection

Infection can be a complication of any wound. It involves the growth of bacteria leading to heat, redness, swelling and pain. An infected limb may be so swollen and painful that it may resemble a broken leg. Infection can spread into the bloodstream, usually causing the cat to run a fever and to go off its food. A very serious infection can end in major surgery or possibly death. A common result of an infection is an abscess, often caused by the bite of another cat. Likely areas for an abscess are the head, legs and base of the tail.

Signs of Infection

- Swelling
- Limping
- Pain
- Colored discharge (usually cream, yellow, green, brown or blood-tinged)
- Foul odor

What to Do

- Transport to your veterinarian (see page 123).

Snake Bites

Most snakes are not poisonous. However, pit vipers (rattlesnakes, copperheads, and water moccasins) are. A pit viper has two fangs that puncture the skin and pump the venom. Coral snakes are also poisonous.

The parts of a cat usually bitten are the head and the legs. If you cannot identify the snake when the cat is bitten and the wound consists of two small openings close together, assume that the snake is poisonous.

A cat bitten by a poisonous snake is in a very serious predicament. The two keys to survival are keeping the cat quiet and obtaining prompt medical attention.

Signs of a Snake Bite

- Two deep punctures

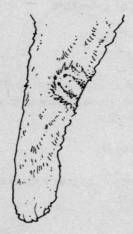

- Swelling
- Area tender and painful to touch
- Weakness
- Wobbling
- Acting nervous

What to Do

- Identify the type of snake, if possible.
- Keep animal quiet.
- Restrict its movement. (This reduces the amount of venom pumped around the body.)
- Apply a tourniquet only if bite is on the lower part of a leg and you think that the snake was poisonous.
    - Wrap a thin belt, bandage or string several times around the leg above the wound.

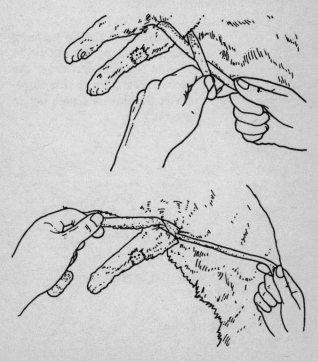

- Tie into a bow.

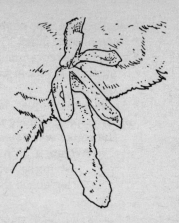

- The tourniquet should be snug but not too tight. You should be able to slip a finger under the tourniquet. (The goal is to restrict the flow of blood, not to stop it.)

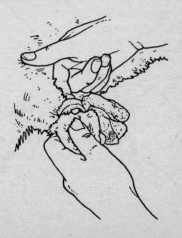

- Keep the cat warm. This reduces the effect of shock.
- Transport to your veterinarian (see page 123). If you cannot reach medical attention within a short period of time, loosen the tourniquet for 60 seconds every 10 minutes.

What NOT to Do

- Do NOT cut the wound and try to suck out the snake venom. This rarely helps and may cause more damage.
- Do NOT apply a tourniquet if the cat resists. Exciting the cat will hasten the spread of the toxins around the body.

Insect Stings

Most insect stings are painful but harmless. However, it is possible that a cat may have an allergic reaction to the insect venom, causing its airway passages to contract. This makes breathing difficult and reduces the effectiveness of the cardiovascular system. The end result can be shock and sometimes death.

Signs of an Insect Sting

- Swelling, usually around the face or legs
- Heat felt when touched
- Possible shock within 30 minutes (if allergic reaction takes place)

What to Do

- Remove stinger, if still in cat.
    - Use tweezers.
    - Grasp stinger at point of entry to skin.

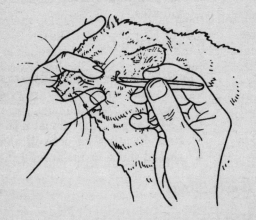

- Pull straight out using a steady, even pressure.
- Apply a cold compress or cloth soaked in cold water.
- Transport to your veterinarian (see page 123).

What NOT to Do

- When removing a stinger, do NOT squeeze the venom sack. This will inject more venom into the cat.

11 Feline Urological Syndrome (FUS) & Blocked Cat

Overview

Feline Urological Syndrome (FUS) is the common term for Lower Urinary Tract Disease. It can be caused by the formation of sand, stones or plugs, urethral infection, bladder infection, cancer of the urethra or bladder, metabolic disorders, congenital abnormalities or any combination of these problems. Cats suffering from FUS can experience pain or irritation when urinating.

Untreated FUS can lead to a blocked cat. This occurs when mucus plugs, sand, grit or small stones (known as calculi) block the urethra and prevent the passing of urine from the bladder. As a result, the bladder backs up and diminishes the kidney's ability to function as the body's filter. This leads to a build up of toxic by-products in the body. The end result is that the cat is poisoned. This problem most commonly appears in young males; females are very rarely blocked. A blocked cat cannot pass urine, can be in a great deal of pain and will often go off its food and water. It is a life-threatening situation that requires immediate medical attention.

The risk of FUS and blockage can be limited by feeding your cat a low ash diet that contains an acidifier. The low ash content reduces the amount of minerals excreted in the urine. The acidifier helps keep the minerals that are excreted in a soluble form. The combination of the two help prevent the formation of sand, grit and stones.

Signs of FUS

- Frequent urination with small amount passed
- Licking at the genitalia
- Blood in urine
- Unusual behavior (such as urinating in uncommon areas of house)
- May eat less than normal

What to Do

- Transport to your veterinarian immediately, if the cat is a male (see page 123). If the cat is definitely a female and not in obvious discomfort, transport to your veterinarian within 24 hours.

Signs of Blocked Cat (almost always a male)

- Frequent crouching and straining to urinate with little or no passing
- Penis sticking out, usually dry and purple in color
- Licking at genitalia
- May cry in pain when picked up
- Lethargic
- Not eating
- Vomiting

- Change in behavior; may be scared and/
  or vicious

What to Do

- Transport to your veterinarian immediately (see page 123). The length of time between blockage and treatment may determine the extent of kidney damage. Serious damage can be fatal.

12   Burns

Overview

A burn is the destruction of tissue by extreme and localized heat. The severity of a burn is measured by how deep the skin is affected and how much surface area is covered. Often the full extent of a burn is not known until several days after the accident.

There are three types of burns.

- Thermal Burns
- Chemical Burns
- Electrical Burns

A thermal burn is the most common. It is caused by being scalded by boiling water, touching an open flame or coming in contact with a hot surface such as an oven door or stovetop. A thermal burn will turn the skin red. It may blister and cause the hair around the burn to be singed.

A chemical burn is caused by the spillage of corrosive materials on the cat. A substance containing an alkali such as lye or ammonia will turn the affected area white or brown and will give the skin a soapy or slippery feel. An acidic substance will cause the skin to dehydrate, contract and darken. Acid burns are very painful, unless the nerve endings have been killed. This would result in no pain but is still very serious.

An electrical burn is discussed in Chapter 13 Electrocution (see page 93).

Signs of Burns

- Skin turning red, white or brown
- Hair singed or falling out in spots

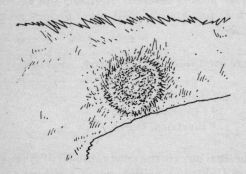

- Skin painful to touch
- Skin contracting
- Skin soapy or slippery to feel
- Blisters

What to Do

- Put on gloves, if available. If you do not wear gloves while treating a chemical burn, you may also be burned.
- Clean and treat burn.

For burns that leave the skin intact

- Wash burned area with water. Use a gentle stream or place in a bath.

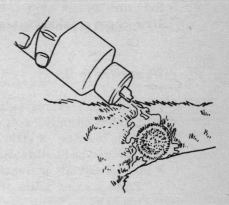

- Put a cold compress on the area burned. (The faster the skin is cooled down, the less damage will occur and the greater the chance for a favorable outcome.)

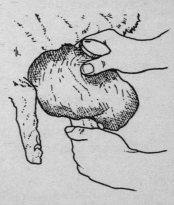

For burns that go through the entire thickness of the skin.

- Cover with dry cloth or towel. (Washing the burn is too painful.)

- Transport to your veterinarian (see page 123).

What NOT to Do

- Do NOT underestimate a burn. It is prone to infection and is easily complicated. A burn covering as little as 15% of the body can be life-threatening.
- Do NOT put oils or creams on the burn. Items such as butter or margarine do not help.

13   Electrocution

Overview

Electrocution occurs when an electrical current passes through the body. It commonly happens when a cat chews through an electrical cord. It can also be caused by being in contact with power lines, touching exposed wires, and being struck by lightening.

There are two problems caused by electrocution. First, the electrical current can create tremendous heat and cause an electrical burn. Second, the current may result in the shut down of key organs such as the heart, the lungs and the kidneys.

The danger of electrocution is deceptive. An animal may appear to recover from a shock within a few minutes. However, the full effects may not appear until 24 to 48 hours after the event. Possible consequences are that the lungs gradually fill with fluid or that the heart may develop an abnormal rhythm. Any cat that has been electrocuted should be examined by a veterinarian.

Electrocution Prevention

Since most electrocution occurs by chewing through electrical cords, kittens that are teething or going through a chewing phase are especially at risk. You can take a few steps to minimize the chance of an accident.

- Unplug cords and equipment not in use.
- Replace old or frayed wires.
- Use a product designed to deter chewing. This is applied directly to an object and has a bitter taste that most cats do not like.

Signs of Electrocution

- Burns, usually around the mouth (most burns will have a pale center surrounded by redness and swelling)
- Convulsions
- Collapsed or lying on side
- Low respiratory rate (under 10 breaths per minute)
- Loss of consciousness
- Heart may have stopped
- Voiding urine and feces

What to Do

- Switch off electrical source.
- Check for vital signs. (Is the cat breathing and does it have a heartbeat?)
- Transport to your veterinarian (see page 123). If your cat does not have any vital signs and proper veterinary care is not available, attempt CPR (see page 51). Even if your cat appears to fully recover, you should take your cat to your clinic immediately.

What NOT to Do

- Do NOT touch the cat if it is still in contact with the electrical current. If you do, you may also be electrocuted. If the cat is touching the source of electricity and is very rigid, it is probably still being shocked. Also watch for any water that may be in contact with the cat.

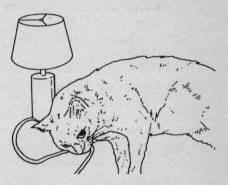

Before touching the cat, turn off the electricity by shutting it off at the source or pulling out the plug (**do not touch any exposed wires**). If you cannot shut off the electricity, move the cat with a non-metal object (such as a broomstick).

14   Heat Stroke

Overview

Cats use the respiratory system to control body temperature. When hot, cats inhale cool air through the nose and exhale hot air through the mouth. The faster cats breathe, the quicker their bodies cool down.

This process works as long as the outside temperature is under the normal 101 to 102.5 degree body temperature of cats. When the outside temperature approaches or exceeds this, a cat cannot efficiently cool itself down. The inability to lose excess body heat can result in heat stroke. This causes a reduction of blood circulation, reduced performance of the kidneys (the blood cleaning filter) and swelling of the brain. It has a high mortality rate.

The most common cause of heat stroke is leaving cats in cars. On a hot day, the temperature in a car can reach 130 degrees in a short period of time. The temperature can soar even if the windows are open. Another cause is keeping a cat in a room without good ventilation or air conditioning. A third is accidentally trapping a cat in a clothes dryer. If a dryer is warm and the door is open, a cat may crawl in for a nap. You can then inadvertently shut the door and start the machine with the cat inside.

The chance of heat stroke can be diminished simply by not leaving a cat in a car during the summer, by keeping a fan or air conditioner on low when it is confined to the home and by checking the clothes dryer before starting it.

Signs of Heat Stroke

- Extreme panting
- Excessive salivation
- Collapse
- Anxious expression on face
- Rectal temperature of 105 degrees or higher

What to Do

- Get the cat's temperature down.
    - Immerse in or hose down with cold water. Keep in water until the temperature goes down.

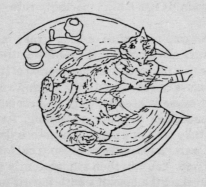

- Or give an alcohol bath.
    - Soak the legs with rubbing alcohol.

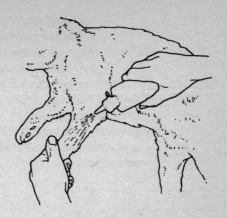

- Pour a small amount on the body.

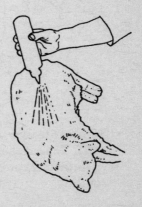

- Place an ice pack on the head and around the body.
- Check the body temperature with a rectal thermometer every 5 minutes. Stop heat reduction when the temperature reaches

103 degrees. (Do not be alarmed
if the temperature drops a few
degrees below normal. A high
temperature is much more
serious than a low one.)
- Give cold water to drink. Allow to drink
  as much as possible.
- Vigorously massage the legs. This helps
  maintain the blood flow and counter-
  acts shock.

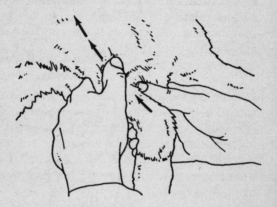

- Transport to your veterinarian (see page
  123). The cat should be examined even
  if its temperature drops back to normal
  quickly.

What NOT to Do

- Do NOT put the cat's head under water
  when immersing it.
- Do NOT put alcohol on the cat's head
  when giving an alcohol bath.

15   Cold Exposure & Frostbite

Overview

Cold exposure (also known as hypothermia) happens when the body temperature becomes much lower than the normal range of 101 to 102.5 degrees. All cats are at risk because of their large body surface relative to their body weight, which facilitates heat loss. Kittens, older cats and injured cats are especially vulnerable. Exposure is very serious and frequently results in death.

In addition, exposure to cold may cause frostbite, a condition in which the skin tissue begins to die. It is possible to develop this condition without suffering serious hypothermia. The parts of a cat prone to frostbite are the tail, tips of the ears and footpads. Frostbitten tissue is very fragile and should be handled very carefully.

The chance of cold exposure and frostbite can be greatly diminished if the cat is brought inside when the temperature falls below freezing or in extreme cold, windy weather.

Signs of Cold Exposure

- Stiff muscles
- Shivering
- Cold to touch
- Dilated and fixed eye pupils

- Low pulse rate (below 150 beats per minutes)
- Low respiratory rate (below 10 breaths per minute)
- Subnormal body temperature

Signs of Frostbite

- Scaling of the skin
- Loss of hair
- White hair
- A leathery-feel to the skin

What to Do

- Handle carefully and very gently.
- Warm cat slowly.
    - Wrap in a blanket.
    - A hot water bottle can be used. Place it underneath the blanket, not directly in contact with the cat.

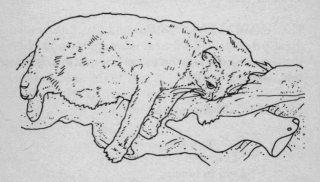

- A hair dryer can be used. Set on warm, not hot.
- Transport to your veterinarian (see page 123). If you cannot reach medical attention quickly, place the cat in a sink or tub of warm water (105-110 degrees). Keep its head above water.

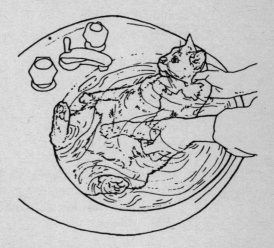

What NOT to Do

- Do NOT warm cat too quickly. Because the blood supply to the skin and limbs has been shut down, hypothermic cats can easily be burned.

16   Choking & Object in Mouth

Overview

Choking occurs when an animal cannot breathe normally due to an object in its throat blocking the airway. Kittens are especially at risk because they often try to swallow the objects that they chew on while teething. These objects can become stuck in the throat, causing the animal to choke. If your cat is choking, you must immediately attempt to dislodge the object blocking the airway; do not wait for veterinary assistance. Choking can be fatal.

It is possible that an object can be stuck in the mouth without causing the animal to choke. While the cat may be able to breathe, the object may shift and subsequently block the airway. Therefore, it is potentially dangerous and should be removed as quickly as possible.

Use care when handling an injured animal. A cat that is choking or has an object stuck in its mouth may panic and can inflict considerable damage. It may lash out or try to bite you when you attempt to remove the object. If you are injured, seek medical attention.

Signs of Choking

- Not able to breathe

- Rubbing face on ground
- Pawing at mouth
- Eyes bulging
- Blue tongue
- Choking sound

What to Do

- Try to remove the object by hand.
    - Hold cat securely. A good method is to wrap it in a thick towel with only the head sticking out.

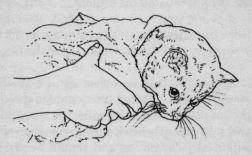

- Open mouth wide.
- Grab object with hand.
- Pull out gently.

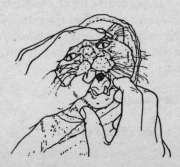

- If unsuccessful, pick up by back legs. Swing back and forth several times.

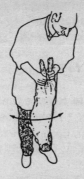

- If unsuccessful, use the Heimlich maneuver. (This forces air out of the lungs and blows the object out of the airway.)
  - Lay cat on side.
  - Place one hand on spine behind the chest.
  - Grasp the lower part of the rib cage with the other hand.

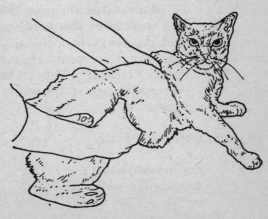

- Using hand on the lower ribs, squeeze in and upward. This action forces air out of lungs and should blow the object out of the throat (too much force may cause internal damage).
  - If object is still stuck, repeat rapidly several times.
- Transport to your veterinarian (see page 123). If that is not possible and the cat has no pulse or respiratory rates, attempt CPR (see page 51).

What NOT to Do

- Do NOT wait for a veterinarian to remove the object blocking the airway. A choking cat cannot breathe and will probably die within a short period of time. You must take action.
- Do NOT assume that the crisis is over when the object is removed. The throat will often swell up when something has been stuck in it. This swelling might block the airway. In addition, internal damage may have occured by use of the Heimlich maneuver. The cat should be examined by your veterinarian as soon as possible.

Signs of Object in Mouth

- Excessive drooling
- Rubbing face on ground

- Pawing at mouth
- Difficulty in swallowing
- Interest in food, but not eating

What to Do

- Try to remove the object by hand. Use the same procedure as with choking (see page 106).
- Transport to your veterinarian (see page 123).

What NOT to Do

- Do NOT force the removal of the object by hand. If it does not come out easily, leave it in place and transport to your veterinarian immediately.
- Do NOT pull out string or thread if part of it has been swallowed. It might saw through the stomach or intestines.
- Do NOT pull out fish hooks or any objects embedded in tissue. This might cause more damage and serious bleeding.
- Do NOT struggle with your cat. If it is uncooperative, take it to your veterinarian.

17   Poison

Overview

A poison is any substance that can cause illness or death if it gets into the body. Most animal poisonings are self-inflicted by ingestion, inhalation, absorption or injection. Two of the most common ways are eating a poisonous house plant and licking off excess flea and tick medicine from the skin.

There are thousands of poisonous substances. As a result, the large variety of symptoms makes diagnosis difficult. Frequently, a veterinarian has to attempt treatment when the type of poison is not known or when it is not certain that the animal has been poisoned. It is important to convey as much information as possible to your doctor.

Generally, you will not see your cat poison itself. You might assume this has happened if your cat is acting in a peculiar manner (especially if it has been missing for a period of time).

If you see your cat eat or come in contact with a poison, take it to your veterinarian immediately. Do not wait until signs of a problem develop.

Poison Prevention

Many cases of poisoning are caused by cats eating something that is around the house. There are several steps that can be taken to prevent this from happening.

- Make a list of all plants in the home and garden.
    - Find out which are poisonous.
    - Remove them or keep them out of reach.
- Never give medication intended for humans, such as aspirin or other pain-relieving products, to your cat.
- Keep all chemicals, cleaning fluids, insecticides, fertilizers, and medicines out of reach. Other common household poisons are antifreeze, mouse and rat poison, roach poison and slug poison.
- Do not overuse medical compounds such as flea and tick products. Always read and follow the instructions carefully.

Signs of Poisoning

- Severe vomiting
- Severe diarrhea
- Shaking
- Convulsions
- Blood in vomit, feces or urine
- Bluish color to tongue
- Weakness
- Collapse
- Difficulty breathing
- Excessive drooling
- Severe irritation of the eyes or mouth
- Peculiar substance on skin or coat

What to Do

- If the poison is on the skin, wash the substance off.
    - Use a lot of water.
    - Wear rubber gloves to avoid poisoning yourself.
- Allow cat to drink as much water as possible. (Water dilutes most poisons.)
- Give activated charcoal tablets, if available. (Charcoal absorbs many poisons.)
- Get a sample of the poison, if possible.
- Get a sample of vomit or stool, if poison not available.
- Transport to your veterinarian (see page 123). Telephone before departing. Your doctor may have special instructions, such as inducing vomiting to limit absorption.

What NOT to Do

- Do NOT wait for signs of poisoning to develop. Take your cat to your veterinarian if you see it ingest or come into contact with a toxic substance.
- Do NOT induce vomiting unless directed to do so by your veterinarian. Many poisons will burn the throat.
- Do NOT give anything by mouth if the cat is convulsing or unconscious.
- Do NOT give any medication such as aspirin or other pain-relieving products

unless directed to do so by your veterinarian.

18   Vomiting & Diarrhea

Overview

Vomiting and diarrhea clean out a cat's gastrointestinal system. The most common cause of vomiting or diarrhea is a sudden change of diet. A cat, accustomed to the effects of a particular food, may suffer an upset stomach if a different type of diet is abruptly introduced. Other causes include intestinal parasites, bacterial infections, motion sickness, internal foreign bodies, kidney failure and poisoning. Vomiting and diarrhea can range from not serious to very serious. With a kitten, any vomiting or diarrhea should be considered serious.

Prevention of Vomiting & Diarrhea

There are a few steps that you can take to eliminate many of the common causes.

- Do NOT feed your cat tablescraps.
- Avoid changing the type of food suddenly.
- Do NOT allow your cat to nibble on house plants.
- Groom your cat everyday to reduce the chance of hairballs.
- Limit access to items that can be swallowed, such as string, yarn and thread.
- Have your veterinarian perform regular fecal checks.

Signs—Not Serious

- Happens only once or twice
- No other signs of problems

What to Do

- Withhold all food for 24 hours.
- Give water.
- If symptoms stop after 24 hours, feed boiled white meat off the bone (chicken or turkey) with boiled white rice for 2 to 3 days. Gradually switch back to regular food.

Signs—Serious

- Symptoms lasting more than 24 hours
- Vomiting or has diarrhea frequently
- Blood in stool or vomit
- Fever
- Evidence of pain
- Weakness or collapse
- Dehydration (eyes sunk in sockets and skin not springing back into place when pinched)
- Signs of other problems (like runny eyes or nose and high respiratory rate)
- Any vomiting and diarrhea by a kitten

What to Do

- Transport to your veterinarian (see page 123).

19   Drowning

Overview

Drowning occurs when the lungs of an animal become flooded with fluid. This stops the inhalation of air and shuts down the respiratory system. Even if a drowning episode does not stop the animal from breathing, it can be serious. Excess fluid can damage the lungs, reducing their ability to absorb oxygen. As a result, a life-threatening situation may exist several hours after the incident occurred.

Drowning is uncommon among cats because they are naturally wary of water. In addition, most are good swimmers over short distances.

Signs of Drowning

- Panic and frantic effort to swim
- Motionless in water

What to Do

- Pull tongue out of mouth.

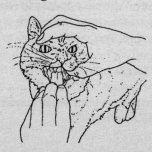

- Drain the water from the lungs.
  - Pick up by hind legs.

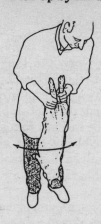

  - Gently swing back and forth until fluid stops coming out.
- Transport to your veterinarian (see page 123). If this is not possible and the cat has no pulse or respiratory rates, attempt CPR (see page 51).

What NOT to Do

- Do NOT assume that the emergency is over if the cat appears to recover. Internal damage to the lungs may have occurred and might lead to secondary flooding over a period of several hours. Or such damage may limit the ability of the lungs to function properly, reducing the amount of oxygen absorbed into the bloodstream.

20   Seizures

Overview

A seizure occurs when a cat appears to lose control
of its body due to a malfunction of the brain. In
controlling the nervous system, the brain acts like
a computer. It stores a massive amount of information and sends messages to the various parts of the
body via electrical impulses. When the brain mal-
functions, the impulses that excite or turn on a body
function may overwhelm those that suppress or
turn off a function. This produces uncontrollable
twitching and erratic behavior. The most common
cause of seizures is epilepsy. However, seizures can
be the result of several other afflictions such as
tumors, hyperthyroidism, meningitis or poisoning.

There are two types of seizures. A general seizure
(or grand mal seizure) affects the entire brain. The
second, partial seizure (also known as a focal seizure or petit mal seizure), only affects a portion of
the brain. However, it can grow to be a general
seizure.

For cats that suffer recurring seizures, medication
may be prescribed. These drugs do not always
prevent seizures, but they help reduce the number
and severity by stabilizing the cell membranes of
the nerves in the brain. If your veterinarian does
prescribe medication, you should give it regularly.
Failure to do so may bring on a seizure.

If your cat has seizures, you should keep a log book. It should record when a seizure takes place and how long it lasts. If you notice that the seizures are occuring more frequently or for longer periods of time, contact your veterinarian within 24 hours.

Signs of a General Seizure

- Lying on side
- Cycling movement of legs
- Rolling of eyes
- Frothing of mouth
- Moving jaw rapidly
- Voiding urine and feces

Signs of a Partial Seizure

- Bumping into objects
- Standing and staring into space
- Trying to catch imaginary flies
- Localized twitching of muscles

What to Do

- Stop animal from hurting itself.

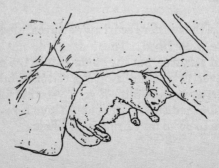

- Move it to a safe area, away from furniture and stairwells.
- Place blankets or pillows around it.
- Time the length of the seizure.

What NOT to Do

- Do NOT put your hand near the cat's mouth.
- Do NOT give anything by mouth.

After the Seizure

- Place cat in a dark room.
- Keep quiet. Do not make any sudden movements or loud noises.
- Give a moderate amount of food and water.
- Wipe away excess saliva.
- Clean up urine and feces.
- Take rectal temperature, if possible.

Contact Your Veterinarian Immediately If....

- It is your cat's first seizure.
- It has more than 1 seizure in a 24-hour period.
- The seizure lasts more than 3 minutes and the cat does not recover quickly and completely. Long, continual seizures can cause death.
- The rectal temperature is over 103.5 degrees.

Contact Your Veterinarian within 24 Hours If....

- The cat is on anti-seizure medication.
- It has a single, short seizure of less than 3 minutes and recovers quickly and completely.

21 Transporting to Your Veterinarian

Overview

Moving a critically injured animal is dangerous; even a slight movement can cause great damage. In addition, an animal in pain may lash out at you. It is crucial that you take precautions to reduce the chance of further injury and to protect both your pet and yourself. If a cat does wound you, seek medical attention.

Things to Remember

- **Support the back**. A seriously injured cat may have a broken back. If the back is not evenly supported when the cat is picked up, a broken bone may pull apart or the ends of the break may rub. This may cut the spinal cord, paralyzing the cat. The back can be supported by sliding a thick towel beneath the cat prior to lifting. If a towel cannot be used, try to keep the back straight when lifting the cat.

- **Keep a broken leg up**. If you suspect that the cat has a broken leg, place it on its side; the damaged limb should be up. This keeps the weight of the body off of the injured leg. You might give the limb some support by placing a folded blanket or towel underneath it.

- **Keep a crushed chest down.** If you suspect that the chest has been crushed, attempt to determine if one side of the chest is in better shape than the other. If this can be done, transport the cat with the least damaged side of the chest up. The lung on that side will function better than the one on the most damaged side. A cat lying with the most damaged side of the chest pointing up may have difficulty breathing. If there is both a broken leg and a crushed chest, the crushed chest should take priority.

Transporting a Cat with Minor Injuries

A cat with minor injuries should be handled in a normal manner. Placing it in a catbox will protect both the cat and you. Use special care not to aggravate the injury. Wrapping the cat in a towel can support an injured limb and help cover a wound. It will also help keep the animal warm, reducing the effects of shock.

Transporting a Cat with Critical Injuries

Most cats can be transported by one person. It is a good idea to slide a towel under the cat and then place both in a cat box. The towel will help support the back while the box will protect both the cat and you. However, do not waste time searching for a towel or a box if they are not readily available.

What to Do

- Position the cat to be picked up.

    - The back is toward you.
    - The side with a broken leg is up. (Place a towel or cloth under the leg for additional support.)
    - The side with a crushed chest is down.

- Slide a folded towel under the cat.
- Slide hands beneath the towel under the cat's body.

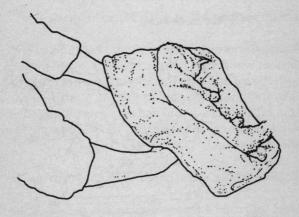

- Pick up using one continuous, fluid motion. Support the back with your hands and forearm.

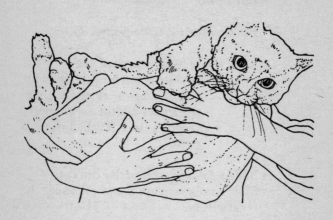

- Place in catbox.

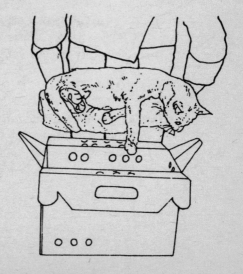

- Walk smoothly to car.

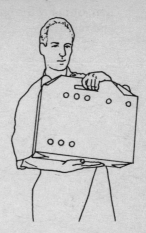

- Place the cat on seat with its back towards the rear of the car.
- Keep warm. (This reduces the effect of shock.)
    - Place a blanket over the cat.
    - Turn on the heater in the car.
- Drive smoothly to your veterinarian.

What NOT to Do

- Do NOT make any sudden movements. The goals are to move the cat as little as possible and to move it smoothly when you must.

PART III

AFTER THE EMERGENCY

22   Giving Medication

Overview

To complete the treatment of your cat, your veterinarian may prescribe medication for you to administer. But the medication serves no purpose if you do not give it in the right dosage at the right times. Your veterinarian will instruct you on when and how to give medication.

Sometimes the prescribed drug will not have the desired effect. In cases such as this, another kind of drug or treatment may be recommended. However, it is impossible to determine the effectiveness of a medication if the instructions are not followed.

Some cats will not allow you to give them medication, despite your best efforts. Care must be taken to avoid being bitten or scratched by an uncooperative, angry animal. If you are injured, you should seek medical attention.

If you are having difficulty giving medicine, contact your veterinarian. You might be advised to use an alternative method or to go to the clinic to have the medicine administered by injection.

Giving Pills

By Hand

- Place your cat on a raised surface so that

it cannot back up. (A table next to a wall works well. Or have someone hold the cat from behind.)
- Open mouth.
    - Place one hand on the cat's muzzle. The thumb is just behind one canine tooth, the index finger behind the other.
    - Pull head back.
    - Other hand pulls the jaw down.

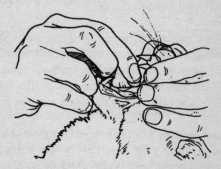

- Drop the pill as far back on the tongue as possible.

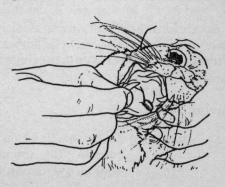

- Touch the pill quickly and gently with the tip of your finger.
- Close mouth.
- Rub the throat until the cat swallows.

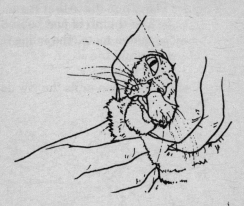

- Open mouth to check if the pill went down. If it did not, repeat.

By Tricking the Cat

- Grind up the pill.
- Mix it in with some food that your cat loves.

Giving Liquid Medication

By Hand

- Open mouth.
    - Place one hand on the cat's muzzle. The thumb is just behind one canine tooth, the

index finger behind the other.
- Keep head level. (Do not tilt back like for pills.)
- Other hand pulls the jaw down.
- Squirt liquid into the side of the mouth. (Do not squirt into the back. The liquid may go down the windpipe instead of the throat.)

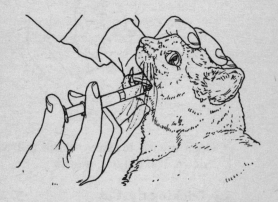

- Close mouth.
- Rub the throat until the cat swallows.
- Open mouth to check if the liquid went down. If not, repeat.

By Tricking the Cat

- Fill a bowl with the cat's favorite food.
- Mix the liquid in thoroughly.

Medicating the Eyes

The common types of medication for the eyes are

ointments and drops. It is important that these come into direct contact with the eyeball.

Ointment

- Clean away any discharge; use a tissue or cotton soaked in warm water.
- Separate the lower eyelid from the eyeball.
    - Hold the cat's head with one hand so that your index finger is on the upper eyelid and the thumb is on the lower eyelid.

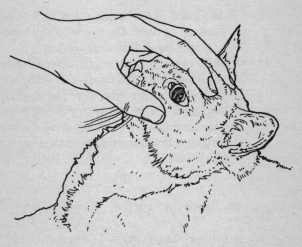

- Move the thumb downward while holding the index finger steady. This creates a small cup between the lower eyelid and the eye.

- Rest the hand holding the tube of ointment on the side of the head.

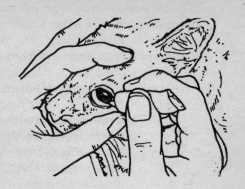

- Run a bead of ointment in the cup. (Use care not to touch the eye with the tube; it might scratch the cornea.)
- Gently close the upper and lower eyelids together. This will cause the ointment to spread a thin film over the eyeball and socket. (Do not worry if the ointment turns white; the eye should clear within a few minutes.)

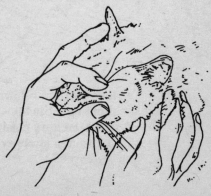

Drops

- Clean away any discharge; use a tissue or cotton soaked in warm water.
- Gently tilt the head back.
- Separate the upper eyelid from the eye-ball.
    - Hold the cat's head with one hand so that your index finger is on the upper eyelid and the thumb is on the lower eyelid.
    - Move the index finger upward while holding the thumb steady.
- Rest the hand holding the eye dropper on the side of the head.

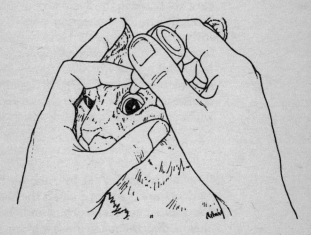

- Place the drops onto the upper portion of the eyeball. (Use care not to touch the eyeball with the dropper; it might scratch the cornea.)

Medicating the Ears

The ear canal of a cat has two sections (vertical and horizontal) with wax glands just in front of the eardrum. It is important that the medication traverses both sections and reaches the eardrum.

- Expose the ear canal by holding up the ear flap.
- Place the ointment or drops in the ear canal.

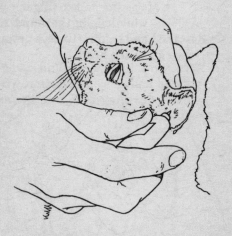

- Massage the ear canal by rubbing the back of the ear where it meets the head. (You may hear a squelch sound. That means that the medicine is making its way down the canal to the eardrum.) Massage for 2 minutes or as long as possible.

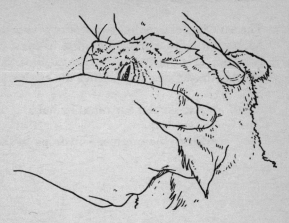

• Wipe away the excess fluid using your finger and a wad of cotton. (Do not insert anything deep into the ear canal.)

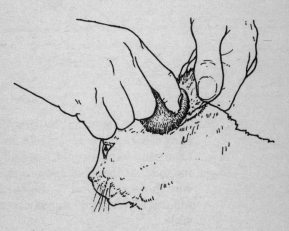

23 Splints, Bandages & Drains

Overview

Splints, bandages and drains are important aids to healing. A splint holds a limb in the correct position so that it can mend. A bandage keeps a wound clean, helps to prevent infection and protects against further injury. A drain is placed in a wound so that excess fluid does not collect. If one of these devices is being used, you should check it often. If you discover any swelling, excessive drainage, foul odors or additional sores, you should contact your veterinarian.

When checking areas of your cat that may be painful, use care to avoid being bitten or scratched. If you are wounded, seek medical attention.

Splints

A splint is used to position a leg to facilitate the healing of broken bones. It has to be snug enough to hold the limb in the correct position. However, it should not be so tight that it restricts the blood circulation, leads to swelling or causes pressure sores. A splints is difficult to place; most cats need to be anesthetized or sedated before one can be applied. Caring for one can also be difficult.

Care of a Splint

- Check top and bottom for swelling 3 times a day. Do this by putting your finger in both the top and bottom of the splint.
  - The top of the splint should be snug but you should be able to insert your finger.

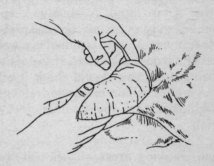

  - You should be able to put your finger between the toes. They should not be cold or swollen.

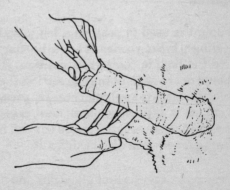

- Check for rubbing and sores 3 times a day.
    - The top of the splint should be able to move slightly when the leg is moved.
    - Your finger should be dry when you pull it out from between the toes. If it is not, there may be open sores draining fluid.
- Keep the splint clean. Put an old sock over it and tape it in place.
- Keep the cat quiet. It is best kept indoors throughout the convalescent period.
- If it chews the splint, put an Elizabethan collar on the cat (see page 147).

Bandages

Bandages keep wounds clean and dry, reducing the chance of infection. They also protect against additional damage.

Care of a Bandage

- Check for swelling and pus around the wound area. These are signs of infection.
- Keep the cat indoors and quiet until healing is complete.
- If it chews the bandage, put an Elizabethan collar on the cat (see page 147).

Drains

Drains are devices that allow pus and excess fluid

to escape from a wound. This aids the healing process. They occasionally need to be cleaned in order to maintain efficiency. Do not be afraid to work with drains; they rarely hurt the cat when manipulated.

There are two common types of drains. A loop drain is a loop of tape that goes through the skin and is closed with a knot.

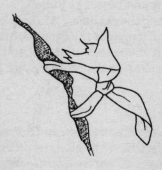

A penrose drain is a short piece of very soft plastic tube placed in the wound. One or both ends of the tube protrude from the skin. The fluid drains around the tube, not through it.

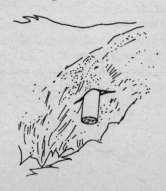

Care of a Drain

- **Prepare the drain for cleaning.**
    - **Loop drains**—Pull the knot to the other end of the incision.

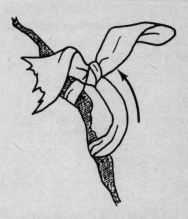

    - **Penrose drains**—Wiggle the end of the drainage tube.

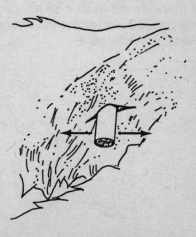

- Remove excess pus and fluid from drainage holes.
  - Soak some gauze with 3% hydrogen peroxide.
  - Dab gauze over drainage holes to loosen dried pus and fluid.
  - Remove pus and fluid.

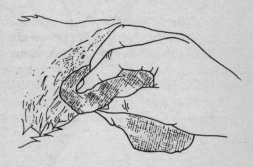

- Clean the drainage holes.
  - Fill eye dropper or syringe with 3% hydrogen peroxide.
  - Squirt a small amount into the holes. (The peroxide will foam up.)

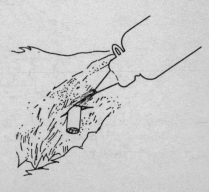

- Dab dry with gauze.
- Repeat 3 times a day or as instructed by your doctor.
- If it chews the drain, put an Elizabethan collar on the cat.

Elizabethan Collar

An Elizabethan collar is a large plastic collar that fits around a cat's neck. It is named after a ruffle that people in England wore in the time of Queen Elizabeth I. It prevents the cat from pawing at its eyes and ears or from chewing at stitches, sores, splints, bandages and drains. Your veterinarian will give you a collar if your cat needs to wear one.

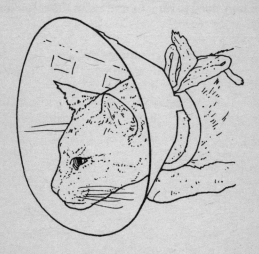

When placing a collar on your cat, fit it just tight enough so that it will not slip over the head. Use a strip of gauze to tie it on.

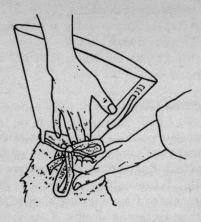

If your cat has had surgery around the face or ears, you may need to remove and clean the collar once a day.

24   Before & After Surgery

Overview

There may be times when it is in your cat's best interest to undergo surgery. In such an instance, there are steps that you can take before and after the operation to help your cat. This chapter gives you some general guidelines. However, some operations require special preparation and care. Your veterinarian will instruct you on the proper action.

BEFORE SURGERY

Preparing Your Cat for Surgery

An operation requires that your cat be given an anesthetic, which exposes it to a slight risk. When anesthetized, a cat loses the protective reflex that closes the windpipe while swallowing. If it were to vomit, a portion may go down the windpipe and into the lungs. This could limit its capacity to breathe and may even result in death. You can help minimize this risk.

What to Do

- No food on the night before surgery.
- No water on the night before surgery. (Very old cats and those with kidney problems should have access to water throughout the night.)

What NOT to Do

• If you do feed your cat on the morning of
  the operation, do NOT hide this fact
  from your doctor. It is better to delay
  surgery than to have a serious problem
  come up while under anesthesia.

AFTER SURGERY

You will need to monitor your cat closely for a
couple of weeks. Doing so will help ensure that it is
healing properly and without complications.

The First 24 Hours

Most surgery takes place in the morning or early
afternoon. The following steps assume that the
operation took place then. Your veterinarian will
give you the instructions on how to care for your cat
during the first 24 hours.

• Do not give food or water until the cat is
  fully awake (usually the morning after
  surgery). Until then, it will still be
  under some of the effects of the anesthesia. Food and water may make it
  vomit.
• Encourage rest. Keep the cat indoors in a
  dark, quiet area.
• Do not touch wound unless instructed to
  do so.
• Do not be alarmed if the wound bleeds a
  small amount. (If there is profuse bleed-

ing, call your veterinarian immediately.)

Until the Stitches Come Out

Stitches normally come out 10 to 14 days after the surgery. The stitches that you can see are usually non-dissolvable; your veterinarian will remove them when appropriate. Stitches beneath the skin are usually dissolvable. They will slowly disappear over the course of several weeks.

Until the stitches are taken out or disappear, you should watch your cat carefully. Its activities should be restricted; if not, the wound may open or tear. This could lead to another operation and a longer period of recovery.

- Keep the cat indoors.
- Do not clean the wound unless instructed to do so.
- Check the wound every day for swelling. It can be the result of several factors.

    - Reaction to stitches—This is the most common cause. The inflamed area does not diminish in size when pressed. And it is usually not too painful or hot to the touch.

    - Organs or tissue extending through incision—Abdominal surgery requires cutting through all of the muscle layers of the abdomen. Stitches that pull muscle layers together sometimes break down or pull apart, allowing abdominal organs and tissue to poke through and form swelling under the skin. If you push this swelling, it will decrease in size. It usually does not feel hot. If a piece of white abdominal fat extends through the skin, do not pull it out; take your cat to your veterinarian immediately.

- Infection—This is often hot to the touch with a thick creamy-colored discharge. The area usually cannot be reduced in size when pushed unless pus comes out between the stitches.

Contact Your Veterinarian If....

- There is any evidence of infection.
- There is any swelling (unless it is obviously caused by the stitches alone).
- There is anything protruding from the wound.
- There is a high body temperature (104 degrees or above).
- The cat is not eating.
- The cat is still very sleepy after 48 hours.
- The cat is vomiting or has diarrhea.

References

AVMA Council on Biologic and Therapeutic Agents. "Canine and Feline Immunization Guidelines." *Journal of the American Veterinary Medical Association* (August 1,1989): 314-317.

Catcott, E.J., DVM, PhD. ed. *Feline Medicine and Surgery, 2nd ed.* Santa Barbara, California: American Veterinary Publications, Inc., 1975.

Ettinger, Stephen J., DVM. *Textbook of Veterinary Internal Medicine: Disease of the Dog and Cat. 2nd ed.* Philadelphia: W.B. Saunders Company, 1983.

Holzworth, Jean, DVM. *Diseases of the Cat: Medicine and Surgery.* Philadelphia: W.B. Saunders Company, 1987.

Kirk, Robert W., DVM, ed. *Current Veterinary Therapy VIII: Small Animal Practice.* Philadelphia: W. B. Saunders Company, 1983.

Kirk, Robert W., DVM, ed. *Current Veterinary Therapy IX: Small Animal Practice.* Philadelphia: W. B. Saunders Company, 1986.

Kirk, Robert W., DVM, ed. *Current Veterinary Therapy X: Small Animal Practice.* Philadelphia: W. B. Saunders Company, 1989.

Kirk, Robert W. DVM. *First Aid for Pets*. New York: E.P. Dutton, 1978.

Kirk, Robert W., DVM and Stephen I. Bistner, DVM. *Handbook of Veterinary Procedures and Emergency Treatment, 4th ed.* Philadelphia: W. B. Saunders, 1895.

Pratt, Paul W., VMD., ed. *Feline Medicine*. Santa Barbara, California: American Veterinary Publications, Inc., 1983.

Sherding, Robert G. DVM., ed. *The Cat Diseases and Clinical Management*. New York: Churchill Livingstone Inc., 1989.

Siegmund, Otto H., et al. eds. *The Merck Veterinary Manual, 5th ed.* Rahway, New Jersey: Merck & Co, Inc., 1979.

Urquhart, G.M., J. Armour, J.L. Duncan, A. M. Dunn and F.W Jennings. *Veterinary Parasitology*. New York: Churchill Livingstone, Inc., 1987.

Index

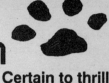
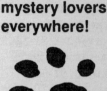